A SUMMARY -GENETICS AND ATHLETICISM

Our height and weight   are influenced by our DNA.   So, how much does our DNA determine our predisposition towards Athleticism?

This short book has been written to attempt to summarise recent scientific material collated over the last decade that discusses the genetic influence on ones athletic ability.

I0468798

Text Copyright ©

First edition: 2016

INTRODUCTION

We have seen numerous athletes over the years that have excelled in their particular field. Many questions arise with such thoughts. Are these athletes predisposed to becoming elite? Is it nature or nurture that makes them the way they are? If it's nature, what genetic makeup aids in their success? Is it a specific type of gene or a select group of genes? If its nurture, again the athlete's environment and upbringing needs to be studied.

The relationship between VO2 max levels and mitochondrial DNA has been a hot research topic lately, with a number of studies trying to delineate the level to which Mitochondria control an individual's maximum oxygen consumption (also called VO2 Max).

Man's quest has always been to achieve more. Nothing ever seems to be enough, and this is particularly true in athletics. "Citius Altius Fortius" goes the saying. It means "Faster, Higher, Stronger" in Latin. How much faster can man go? How much stronger can a human being get?

When it comes to individual athletic prowess, there are some who are better at sprinting, and others who are better at endurance, and so on. What are the factors that distinguish them? Some evidence indicates there are clear biochemical factors at play, which hard wire an individual's VO2max, their lactate threshold, and functional threshold. Are these parameters genetically controlled or are they trainable, and if so by how much?

According to the latest research, there are 23 polymorphisms in genes that play a very crucial role in one's sporting ability. What are they? Why are West Africans better at sprinting and endurance? Can genetic testing determine which individual will be good at certain sports? Is it fair to choose "sports persons" based on genetic testing?

Further, can these tests also determine who is prone to injury? We will try to answer, or at least debate, some of the above questions and a few more in this book.

OXIDATION OF FUEL

We need energy to run our bodies. The fuel for this energy comes from aerobic respiration, which means respiration that requires oxygen. We cannot live without this constant supply of energy. That is exactly why we breathe.

So, what is oxidation of fuel? This means the burning or combustion of carbohydrates and fats in the presence of oxygen. This burning results in the release of molecules "Adenosine Tri Phosphate" or ATP, in short. ATP is the energy we are talking about.

There are two ways in which ATP is released. One is, as mentioned above, in the presence of oxygen. The other is, in the absence of oxygen, also known as anaerobic respiration. The difference between the two is that aerobic respiration, though slower in the release of ATP, is sustained by the constant supply of oxygen by our breathing. Anaerobic respiration is not sustained for long, even though it releases ATP fast.

Where in our body does this oxidation of fuel happen? Our body is made of numerous small cells. Each cell contains organelles of its own. One of the cell's organelle, called the Mitochondria, is responsible for oxidation or aerobic energy production.

GENETICS OF MITOCHONDRIA

The nucleus is one organ of the cell which contains chromosomes. The chromosomes contain DNA, and genes are a part of our DNA. Most of our genes are present in the nucleus. But there is another organ in the cell, called the mitochondria, which has its own set of genes. The role of these genes has recently come to light.

In all, the mitochondria contain about 37 genes. They are just a small fraction of the genes of our body. Nevertheless, they are very important, specifically to aiding athleticism. The mitochondrial genes are highly prone to mutations. These mutations or changes could influence our lives tremendously. As mentioned above, respiration and oxidation depend upon mitochondria. Hence, these genes form the base of an athlete's life. It's inheritance could play a role in shaping the future of a sports star.

MATERNAL INHERITANCE OF MITOCHONDRIAL DNA

There is a reason why the mitochondrial DNA is passed on only from the mothers and not the fathers. Both the sperm and the egg contain mitochondria. The sperm consists of three parts, being the head, the body, and the tail. Mitochondria are present only in the body part of the sperm. During fertilisation, only the head of the sperm fuses with the egg and hence the mitochondria are lost with the body. The fertilised zygote contains only the mitochondria from the maternal egg. In short, the mother can pass on her mitochondria to her sons and daughters, but only the daughters can pass it on further. The mitochondria of the sons do not pass on any further.

MITOCHONDRIA AND ATHLETISM

How does mitochondria relate to exercise and endurance? Since mitochondria releases energy in the form of ATP, we can say that the more we exercise, the more energy we need. The more energy we need, the more that needs to be produced. It's a cycle, hence the old sporting term: "Train your Mitochondria".

The process by which the mitochondrial density increases is called "Mitochondrial Biogenesis". To stimulate this biogenesis, the body requires the functioning of two signals concurrently.   One such signal is the calcium concentration in the skeletal muscle cells. An increase in calcium due to muscle contraction releases an enzyme called Calcium Calmodulin Kinase (CAMK). The other signal required is the reduction of high energy phosphates such as phosphocreatinine and ATP. This happens automatically during high intensity exercise when the process of aerobic respiration is not able to maintain their levels. These signals release another enzyme called 5' AMP Activated Protein Kinase (AMPK). Both CAMK and AMPK are closely related, and together, they help in the production of proteins required for mitochondrial biogenesis.(1).

As a practical example, it is easier to explain this process. A high intensity exercise session of short duration (30 minutes) produces the same amount of ATP as a low intensity exercise of longer duration. For mitochondrial biogenesis to happen, a particular amount of ATP needs to be produced and released. This also means that you need to exercise above your capacity to produce ATP and therefore, energy. If you exercise at or below your capacity, no mitochondrial biogenesis will take place. Since mitochondria is responsible for all the energy production and respiration, the DNA present in mitochondria is examined to find out changes in its genetic makeup that could lead to differences in people with respect to fitness and VO2 max levels. (2)

THE ROLE OF VO2 MAX

As already mentioned, VO2 max means maximum oxygen consumption. That is, the amount of oxygen a person can inhale. When you exercise, the amount of oxygen you inhale and the carbon dioxide you exhale increases. But beyond a limit, it does not increase. This limit is the maximum level and is called VO2 max.

Research says that the greater a person's VO2 max, the greater will be his   or her endurance capacity.   Many sporting communities around the world use this test as a broad-brush indicator to ones potential.   It is measured in ml/kg/min, i.e., millilitres per kilogram of body weight per minute.

What is the VO2 max of individuals normally? These values differ between men and women.   For women between the ages of 20-29, VO2 max values from 33.0 to 36.9 is considered good. Values between 37 and 41 are excellent and those greater than 41 are superior.

For men between the ages of 20-29, VO2 max values from 42.5 to 46.4 is considered good, 46.5-52.4 is excellent, and those above 52.4 is superior.   Lance Armstong, a cyclist has a value of 84.0 whereas Bjorn Daehlie, a cross country skier, has value of 90. You can now understand how they have such endurance capacities.

RELATIONSHIP BETWEEN VO2MAX AND GENETICS

A recent study was conducted to estimate the relationship that VO2 max has with one's genetics. Groups of people in different age ranges were subjected to sports related training programs. The type of training was the same for all the groups. The time duration also did not differ.   Despite this, it was found that the increase in VO2 max between the different groups was not the same.

The gene coding for the Angiotensin Converting Enzyme (ACE) was studied. This was studied because it plays an important role in the cardiovascular system.   It helps in generating angiotensin from its precursors. This hormone also helps in vasoconstriction. It is currently the target of many drugs developed by the pharmaceutical companies.

Before we go into any details about the research, we'll explain a bit about the genetics of the ACE gene.   Each individual contains two genes for each enzyme; One they inherit from their father, the other from their mother. In case of ACE, there is an 'I' form of the gene and a 'D' form. So an individual can be either an II type, DD type or an ID type depending upon which they inherit from both their parents.

It has been found that those people with DD type have high VO2 max levels. Those with the II type have the lowest levels and the ID type have levels in between the other two. 50% of the people belong to the ID group and 25% each to both II and DD types.

One study was conducted on 724 people who previously led very sedentary lives. They were given a training program which included a fitness and exercise regimen for about 20 weeks. At the end of the 20 weeks, their VO2 max levels were checked again. Their results were concordant with the above genotype differences.

The DD genotype showed an increase of 2.6-2.7 L/min of VO2

max. The II and ID type showed an increase of only 400-480 ml/min (4). So this study indicates some individuals appear to have a much greater capacity to train their VO2 max (5).

Another study was conducted on some postmenopausal women who led a regularly active lifestyle. Women who had the same age, physical activity level, and body type participated. Even though differences were seen with respect to the genotypes, in this study the VO2 max levels of the ACE II type showed a higher increase. But there was a reason for this, and once the reason was neutralised, the study showed a similar difference between the genotypes. (6)

Even though these studies show a difference in VO2 max levels based on individual genotypes, it still cannot be confirmed whether genes are the only reason for such a difference. This is because each study had its limitations under which it was conducted.

The other issues that need to be potentially considered are:

- Whether different genes were the only reason for such a difference or were there other factors involved.

- Can the VO2 max level be achieved by all people just by good training, regardless of their genotypes?

- Is VO2 max associated with other genes which may also be a contributing factor?

- Once the human genome project is completed, other genes that could be linked to VO2 max can also be studied.

BIOLOGY BEHIND THE ACE GENE

The Angiotensin Converting Enzyme (ACE) produces active angiotensin from its precursor. Basically, this enzyme cleaves angiotensin I, which is the inactive precursor. This leads to the production of angiotensin II which is the active form.

Angiotensin II has many uses in our body. One of them relates to its role during any physical activity. Angiotensin II constricts the arteries and increases the blood pressure of the individual. It also helps in stimulating the thirst centres of the brain. This in turn indirectly raises blood pressure and blood volume. Once this happens, the kidneys start preserving more water.

The D type of ACE gene, which is present in sprint athletes, has higher amounts of angiotensin II levels. This leads to increased muscle strength. This increase in muscle strength and mass, along with higher amounts of the fast muscle fibres, allows sprint athletes to excel in their fields.

Note: The 'D' allele of the ACE gene refers to the deletion of a short segment of the gene. Thus, individuals who inherit the 'D' allele from both their parents come under the 'DD' category.

VO2MAX AND MITOCHONDRIA

The relationship between VO2 max levels and mitochondrial DNA has been a focal research topic lately, with a number of studies trying to delineate the level to which Mitochondria control an individuals VO2max. In one such study, 46 sedentary people were given a 20 week training program involving endurance exercises. It was found that some people showed a lower response to the training program and their VO2 max levels did not increase much. These people were found to have a polymorphism in a gene encoding a subunit of NADH dehydrogenase enzyme. NADH dehydrogenase is directly related to mitochondria and fitness because it is responsible for the respiration and energy production which mitochondria performs.

Next, the frequency of the presence of this polymorphism was tested in the different groups. No difference was observed in the frequency levels. This could be because all the individuals in this study had the same origin. Possibly if they had a different ancestry, the frequency would have been different.

A similar study was conducted in China, though the subjects of this study were chosen differently. There were three groups of people, which were segregated as elite endurance athletes, general endurance athletes, and sedentary individuals. Approximately nine polymorphisms were found, and they had different frequency levels in the different groups. This time, their ethnicity was well defined. But the researchers in this case were not sure if VO2 max was responsible for this polymorphism, or if other factors related to endurance were also involved. Since some studies found a difference in the frequencies and some did not, there is some disagreement within the scientific community. More research needs to be done to find out if less oxygen is supplied to the muscles of those with less endurance, or their muscles do not utilise the available oxygen adequately.(2)

THE ROLE OF ACTN3 GENOTYPE

Endurance and power are two things which any sports person needs. Some need one more than the other depending on the sport, some might need both in equal measures. Which gene is responsible for which feature needs to be elucidated.

Many genes are responsible for stamina and power in an individual, therefore known as a polygenic trait (meaning many genes contribute to a single factor or trait). Many genes and their variants have been associated with stamina and endurance, but only a few have given consistent results. The ACE gene, as mentioned above is one of them. The other is the ACTN3 gene.

ACTN3 stands for α-actinin-3 gene. This gene has shown consistent results in different groups of sportspersons. Now similar to the ace gene the ACTN3 is split into different genotypes RR, RX and XX. The slow muscle fibres help in slow, yet continuous muscle contractions which are needed for endurance. The fast muscle fibre is responsible for powerful contractions which are needed for sprinting.

The XX genotype group don't have powerful contractions and such people will not be good at sprint events, though they will excel at endurance related events such as marathons (7).

ESTIMATION OF ELITE ATHLETES

Since more than 20 polymorphisms have been identified and in some way shape or form linked to athleticism, can people have all the polymorphisms? How does athleticism depend on these polymorphisms? Does it depend on the number of polymorphisms they have? How varied is the frequency of such polymorphisms?

Based upon mathematical calculations, scientists have tried to estimate if a perfect genetic profile for elite athletes exists, naturally though, this does depend upon the sporting genre. When we take one polymorphism into consideration, it is seen that there is around an approximately 21% chance that an individual will possess a singular "sporting" genotype. If we include a second gene, the frequency of that genotype decreases to a mere 4%. As more and more genes are taken into consideration, the frequency of finding an individual with all these genes decreases exponentially.

In-fact when all 23 polymorphisms were taken into consideration and the frequency was calculated, it was found to be 8.2×10^{-14}%. This means that the probability that an individual can have all 23 polymorphisms in his/her genetic profile is 1 in 1212 trillion.

This equates to there being about a 0.0005% (approx. 1 in 200,000) chance of one individual on the planet having all the 23 polymorphisms. Thus looking at the above statistics, you can realise that there is really no chance of finding an individual who has all 23 polymorphisms, or even 22 or 21.

Due to the polygenic nature of athletic performance, it is difficult to correctly identify the exact nature of power or endurance performance. The difference between the upper and lower limits is quite narrow. It is easy to conclude that a 'perfect' individual is next to impossible.

TOTAL GENOTYPIC SCORE (TGS)

The science of genetics is quite complex. There is a way to determine the genetic potential of an individual. It is estimated using the Total Genotypic Score, or TGS, which has a range between 0-100. When this method was devised, it was thought that an individual having a TGS score of greater than 90 would be considered an elite athlete. However, looking at the above statistics, this has been nullified and scientists are not able to determine what would be the limit of a TGS score to find out if a person is an elite athlete or not. (8)

ETHINICITY AND GEOGRAPHICAL LOCATION

Ethnic diversity and geographical location play a huge role in one's life. It plays a large role in genetics and sports as well. Many a times, you will notice that a particular country or a community dominates certain sports events for generations. There may be world record holders from very small countries, whereas people from some of the bigger and better known countries would not be able to make a mark. This is because there are variations in the frequencies of genotypes of people in different geographical locations or ethnicities.

For example, athletes belonging to north and east Africa are statistically better at endurance events, while hose from West Africa are good at sprint events. People belonging to the Oceanic region have a higher frequency of ACE II polymorphism than the rest of Europe. The Kenyans, Ethiopians, and Moroccans have a higher frequency of genotypes which favour endurance. (9)

POWER - THE SPRINTERS

Jamaicans and West Africans have a long standing history of holding world records in sprinting (Usain Bolt). Reasons have been found for such dominance. For one, they do have D variants of the ACE gene which has been proven to give athletes power and speed. This results in the fast twitch muscles working extremely fast, and their heart is able to pump highly oxygenated blood faster into their muscles. The frequency of this gene is higher in West Africans than in European and Asian populations. In Jamaicans, it is found to be slightly higher than in West Africans.

They also have an abundance of the sports gene ACTN3, which helps them generate powerful muscle contractions . The desirable variant of this gene, R577X, has been found in 75% of Jamaicans and only in 70% of Americans. This is with respect to the entire population of Jamaican and America, not just athletes. There is another peculiar advantage that the Jamaicans have. Jamaica has huge deposits of Aluminium ore. It is a well known fact that the presence of aluminium in the diet can alter a gene's expression. The food grown in the bauxite-rich soil of Jamaica does have a large amount of aluminium in the loam. Aluminium helps in the growth of the fast-twitch muscle fibres in a growing fetus. The number of fast twitch muscles fibres that a person will have is determined in its first three months as a fetus. It does not change after that. This is also another reason why Jamaicans have more fast twitch muscles.

There are some other biological factors which aid Usain Bolt's speed. He can reportedly reach speeds up to 43 km/h, his long legs give him an advantage of 20 cm per stride over the others, and he can complete a race in 40 steps whereas his closest rivals take 44. He is also very symmetrical, which is good for even sprinting. Some 80% of his muscle fibres are of the fast twitch type. A normal human has only 50%. (11)

ENDURANCE ATHLETES

Eero Mantyranta was a famous cross country skier who won 7 Olympic medals. He was supposedly one of the best endurance athletes to have ever graced the planet, and won the 1964 winter Olympic Games by a huge margin.

Many years after his famous victories, scientists had conducted genetic tests on him. A rare mutation was found in the gene responsible for producing the EPO hormone. His body was found to be over-responsive to this hormone which led to the production of more red blood cells. This meant that his blood could carry more oxygen to his heart. This excess capacity for carrying oxygen gave him his endurance power. This mutation was found in his entire family.

This kind of a mutation is very rare. Luckily, just as we have favourable genotypes, we do not have any unfavourable genotypes. If unfavourable genotypes did exist, the mortality rate of people due to lack of fitness activities could well be very high. It is just that some people are good at it, while others are not. (12)

THE 10,000 HOUR THEORY?

Some literature suggests that anyone that anybody can become an elite performer if they practice enough. According to the theory, 10,000 hours of practice, almost equal to 10 years, will make any ordinary person an elite athlete. This has provoked a lot of discussion.

Scientists studied the biographies of around 26 elite sprint athletes, which included Olympic and world champions. The first thing they came to realise was that many of the athletes achieved their world class status in less than five years. This trashed the 10 years and 10,000 hours theory proposed by previous researchers.

The second big finding was that these sprinters were found to be faster than normal, even before they received any training. Their first competitive performance was found to be better than 95% of the rest of the people in the same category. This is true for any sport. The fact that a child is good at something can be identified very early, and they show signs of dominance from their very first event (10).

One athlete, named Abebe Bekela, had won the marathon in the 1960 Rome Olympics. This was famous not just because he won, but because he never had any experience, didn't have a coach, and ran without shoes and still won the gold! This is a very strong example proving that genetic predisposition is a key trait to becoming an elite athlete. (14)

THE SPORTS GENE

David Epstein, the author of the popular book "The Sports Gene", has written very strongly in favour of how genes play a role in elite athletes. Some of the points from his famous book are as follows:

- Some people are slow because of their slow twitch muscle fibres. They cannot become fast by training no matter how hard they try. Thus, nurture will not help them since nature made them the way they are.

- The same mutation in the gene that causes red headedness in people also gives them more tolerance towards pain.

- While playing a game like baseball, having a genetic make up for good eyes is more important than the reaction time. This is because it is the eyes that first judge where the ball is coming from.

- 10% of people having a European ancestry have been found to have a gene mutation which does not let them test positive in spite of being injected with testosterone.

- Short marathoners are more successful than tall ones. This is because, when the body reaches 104 degrees while running, it becomes slow. However shorter athletes don't hit those internal temperatures because they have a larger surface area as compared to their volume.

- Majority of the endurance runners from Kenya come from one particular community called the Kalenjin. Only 12% of Kenyans are Kalenjins, but most of their elite endurance athletes are Kalenjins. Thus, not all Kenyans are good at running marathons.

- The Kalenjins are so good because their genetic makeup allows them to have a large lung capacity, long legs, and lighter limbs.Strong will power is also linked to genes.

- The fact that you get better with practice is also related to genes. Only if you have the genes for it will you be able to do it right.

- Having a good body type for particular sports was also important to succeed.(13)

LACTATE THRESHOLD

Also known as the anaerobic threshold. When you start any physical activity, you will reach a point where you start losing energy, your muscles won't contract as much as they were, and you might start feeling pain and be eventually forced to stop. Just before you start losing energy, lactic acid begins to accumulate. This leads to slowing down of other factors like muscle contraction and energy. The heart rate and running speed at which point lactic acid begins to accumulate is called the lactate threshold.

Lactate threshold is used to determine the fitness level of an individual. It is a better test because it is very sensitive. The greater the lactate threshold of a person, the higher his or her endurance capacity is. Thus, elite endurance athletes will have a very high lactate threshold as compared to sprint athletes or non-sports people. To calculate the lactate threshold of a person, a VO2 max test is done during which time the lactic acid levels of a person is constantly tested. The threshold is the point where accumulation of lactic acid leads to a decline in the performance.The values of lactate threshold depend on both genetics and training (15).

A gene called MCT-1, which is present on the first chromosome of human beings, has been linked to lactate threshold. This gene helps in the production of a protein which transports lactate into the muscles of an individual. The lactate threshold is also linked to the ACE gene, which also influences VO2 max levels (16).

The reason behind this improved performance is that beyond the lactate threshold, a person feels tired and stressed. The muscles and heart are doing their work under stress. Continuous training at this level will lead to the muscles and heart getting used to this stress and working better. So after some time, the level at which you get tired will increase. This simply means that you have improved your endurance.

The other way to improve your lactate threshold is by doing intense short interval training. This means that you do some intense workout for 2-3 minutes, depending on your capacity and give a break in between for 1-2 minutes, before resuming the activity. The break is necessary because a very intense activity cannot be prolonged for a long time. The break is also a recovery period which allows the lactic acid that has accumulated in the skeletal muscles to diffuse out, and then the intense activity can be started again. This kind of interval training has been found to increase the lactate threshold among individuals.

The specificity of the lactate threshold is an important point to be taken into consideration. Lactate threshold is very specific to a particular activity. An individual's lactate threshold for one activity will not be the same for another activity. For example, a cyclist has reached a certain level of lactate threshold by practicing regularly. If you measure his or her threshold level while rowing, you will find it to be generally lower. This is because different muscles are used for both the activities (17).

LUNG CAPACITY AND MICHAEL PHELPS

Lung capacity refers to the amount of oxygen a person can inhale. VO2 max refers to the amount of inhaled oxygen a person can use. VO2 is also referred to as oxygen capacity. This means the higher the lung capacity of a person, the higher his or her VO2 max will be. However, no particular gene has yet been linked to lung capacity.

There are however other factors which can reduce oxygen capacity, thereby making lung capacity inefficient. There are nominally two ways for this to happen. One is that all the inhaled oxygen is not transported to the muscle tissues by the heart or lungs. If your heart does not pump blood up to its capacity, not enough blood will not reach the muscles. This means that the muscles do not receive enough oxygen since blood carries oxygen to all parts of the body. Since the muscles don't receive enough oxygen, the mitochondria don't generate sufficient energy.

The other way of oxygen capacity being reduced is by the lungs. If they are not utilising the oxygen that is coming from the heart or lungs there will not be enough mitochondria in the muscles to utilise the oxygen and burn it into energy.

There are ways to improve lung and oxygen capacity. Although if you are genetically inclined to have low capacity, there is probably only so much that you can do.

There are a few people who have an abnormally high lung capacity. It gives them an unusually high capability of doing any kind of physical exercise (18). Michael Phelps, one of the greatest Olympic swimmers of all time, is one of them. His lung capacity is 12 litres, which is double that of an average individual. This capacity alone gives him a huge advantage over the others in his field.

Phelps' muscles also produce 50% less lactic acid than many other athletes. As we have already discussed, this gives him enormous power and endurance. The width of his arms is greater than his height. He has a arm width on 6'7" whereas his height is only 6'4". His legs are very short as compared to his long trunk or upper body. This trunk is the engine which powers his huge arms and helps him swim faster. These advantages, along with his genes, make him one of the fastest swimmers on earth (19).

PAULA RADCLIFFE

Paula Radcliffe is the fastest marathoner in women's history. Her world record, set more than a decade ago, has not come even close to being beaten. Her record has been a full 3 minutes ahead of the next timing so far.

When she was tested at the age of 17, it was noted that her VO2 max levels were that of an elite athlete rarely seen at that age. It was as high as the level could get in women. She had the ability to withstand high levels of pain, as well. According to what her coaches said, they have never seen anyone being able to bear the kind of pain. According to Radcliffe herself, her body was able to absorb the effect of high intensity training and pain better than others. She definitely had far greater energy and power than most female athletes.

But genetics cannot take away the hard work that an athlete has to do to reach the top. Paula has worked just as hard, if not harder than the others. She had an unrelenting daily and weekly schedule which she would follow no matter what. Of course, her body gave her the ability to do so, but mental strength is another matter altogether. Paula also had the foresight that was somehow genetically better than others. At a time, when she was at the peak of her career, making a biological passport was not possible. However, she asked the authorities to store her samples so that they could be tested when the technology became available. She would also ask for her blood and urine samples to be tested frequently so that her biology could be monitored closely.

Her performance was met with a lot of scrutiny. She had survived every test with flying colours, meaning there was not even a trace of doping found. The queen of the 26.2 miles event will be known as one of the greatest ever (20).

FEMALE ATHLETES AND THE GENDER TRAP

Also known as the Complete Androgen Insensitivity Syndrome. Caster Semenya, from South Africa, is a good example example of such a case. The 18 year old 800 m Olympic gold medalist was stripped of her medal following a gender test, after which she was declared a 'male.' Since she was a 'male,' it meant she had an undue advantage over her female participants. She would be producing male hormones which would give her greater strength and endurance.

This led a young Indian athlete Santhi Soundarajan to attempt suicide after she was told that she failed a gender test. She too was stripped off her 800 m silver medal in the Asian games.(21) Approximately 1% of people in the world are born with such a condition. Such individuals may have characteristics of both male and female. Sometimes it is obvious, at other times, it is not. If such an abnormality is not visible at birth, it may come to be known at other times in a person's life. For example, at puberty, if a girl does not start her menstrual cycles. It may also come to light when a woman is trying to have a baby and is not successful. In a few cases, it comes out when they are competing at high level sports events, like in the case of Caster and Santhi (22).

Stella Walsh was one of the first athletes known to fall into the gender trap. She was one of the fastest sprinters during the 1930s. Luckily for her, her situation came to light only during her death when an autopsy was conducted on her. She was shot at by gunmen about 44 years after her Olympic victory in 1932. Walsh had a rare condition called mosaicism, in which she had mixed chromosomes; Both for male and female. This happens when some cells of her body had male chromosomes and some had female. This led to her having undeveloped male and female organs.

There is a story of Hitler sending a transgender athlete to the 1936 Berlin Olympics, knowing fully well that the person was transgendered. He preferred this athlete over a naturally born female as the results would be better and they would be able to win more medals. How far this story is true is not known. Genetic testing has definitely led to a more dignified way of gender testing (23).

GENE DOPING IN SPORTS

Gene doping can be rightly explained by the definition that the World Anti Doping Agency (WADA) has given for the term. It is defined as "the non-therapeutic use of genes, genetic elements and/or cells that have the capacity to enhance athletic performance". Until recently, genes were used for therapeutic purposes to treat illnesses or diseases. Now, they can be used in healthy individuals to increase performance (24).

The line between gene therapy and gene doping in very thin, as gene doping has evolved from gene therapy. The techniques which were used to treat anaemia and peripheral vascular diseases are the ones being employed for doping as well. This is because the same genes and their enzymes, which are deficient in diseased individuals, are needed to enhance performance in elite athletes.

Generally there are two types of gene doping; One is on the somatic cells, these cannot be inherited, i.e. they cannot be passed on from one generation to the next. The other is on the germline cells. These cells are present in the males sperm and females eggs, or in the embryo. Any genetic change made to these cells can be inherited. Due to ethical issues, genetic research on gene therapy has been banned in germline cells. Therefore, the majority of doping occurs on the somatic cells.

More than 200 genes have in some way been linked to athletic performance and, as explained previously, 20 are very well known and proven. Scientists still do not know the role each gene plays. To avoid risks, they are trying to tweak genes which have a known function in the body. One such gene is the IGF-1 gene. IGF-1 stands for Insulin like Growth Factor-1. This gene helps in bulking up muscles and also repairing damaged ones.

Immunogenicity for pharmaceuticals is indeed very complicated, with many scientific groups working on genes responsible for the release of Erythropoietin (EPO). EPO raises the number of Red Blood Cells (RBCs) in the body thereby supplying more oxygen. EPO, as a drug is famous for its misuse by athletes. Lance Armstrong was one famous athlete who used synthetic EPO often to improve his cycling performances.   Bjarne Riis, also known as Mr. 60%, admitted that he won the 1996 Tour de France using EPO.

TRANSFER OF GENES

How does this happen? How can genes be transferred from one organism to another? Scientists use what are known as vectors to transfer genes. Just like when a mosquito causes malaria in humans, it is known as a vector or carrier. Similarly, to transfer genes, viruses are used as vectors. This is because the virus can transfer their genetic content directly into humans. However, viruses contain harmful or infectious content, which is first cut off or removed from its genome. The human gene of interest is inserted into the virus. The virus is finally injected into humans. This method can also be done using bacteria. Bacteria have a circular DNA in them called a plasmid. Just like a virus, the desired human gene can be put into the plasmid. The bacteria can also be injected into humans. Once the genes are inside, they will start producing the required chemical or enzyme.

However easy it sounds, this technique is dangerous. The bacteria and virus can attack the cells in any part of our body, or it may not necessarily reach the desired cells. This can lead to a different modification in the body than the one desired. It can also be fatal or cause diseases like cancer. There are various ways of targeted delivery of genes into the body, however there will always be risks present.

Most harboured techniques have been developed to treat genetic diseases in humans, though one could argue with limited success. The other point to note is gene doping really is at the forefront of, pushing the boundaries of current technology and scientific understanding, this makes it firstly hard to quantify the frequency of cases, and secondly difficult to trace.

The 34.4-kD glycoprotein hormone was subsequently identified as the humoral regulator of red blood cell production. Decreased tissue oxygen tension modulates EPO levels by increasing expression of the "EPO Gene". To provide some context into the dangers of gene doping, let's look at one example. It was transferred into monkeys and the effect was tested to iterate that the EPO gene increases the amount of red blood cells in the body to improve oxygen uptake. In our body, when oxygen is low, the EPO genes increases RBCs and then switches off when there is enough oxygen. But imagine what will happen when you artificially inject the gene. The EPO gene will constantly produce red blood cells without stopping or switching off. This was because their RBCs had increased so much that blood had to be removed from their bodies to avoid a stroke; Consequentially, the monkeys which were being tested   subsequently died.

Cancer is a serious side effect of such a technology. Cancer is nothing but uncontrolled increase of the cells. If you insert a gene in the body which is meant to boost cell growth and it is not controlled, you would face a similar situation to the monkeys above. The cells will grow uncontrollably, eventually causing a cancer of types. There is also a high risk of immune reactions as well.   The body may kill the virus or bacteria entering into it. In some cases, this immune system shock can kill.

Notably, the technology does not yet exist to remove a gene, so it's a very dangerous game as once the gene is inserted into the body, it cannot be removed and if it does not work, the person will likely not survive (25).

Very soon, ways of detecting gene doping may be identified. Notably, the laws around this are also a bit hazy ; at the time of this publication the author believes there are no laws enforced in "sport" prohibiting gene doping.

GENETIC TESTING TO PREDICT SPORTING ABILITY IN CHILDREN?

We have spoken a lot about how certain genes are involved in the sporting success of an athlete. It raises a big question, can the sporting ability of a child be predicted? Can genetic testing determine whether a person will excel in sport?

The current research in the field points to two key genes, namely ACTN3 and ACE, which have been the most closely linked to athleticism thus far (26). Does this mean in the future sports scholarships or football team selection may be based up a set of specific genes?

Even though science in the area is advancing rapidly, it is still difficult for scientists to analyse genetic results in a way that could predict sporting ability (28).

Facilities like GeneSmart have been set up to look into the issue. There are certain companies which offer testing for up to 10 genes. But they don't reveal exactly what DNA stretches or sequences they are looking into. Some even offer do it yourself kits.

The technology is advancing day by day. All you need is your saliva to do the genetic test. The costs are also coming down rapidly, though it might cost a person between $100 and $200 to do the test. Whole genome sequencing can be done in a day now. But the validity and integrity of such tests is still worth questioning (27).

There are ethical issues involved too. The results of this test can be easily misunderstood and misinterpreted. It is easy for the test results to be used and abused. Also, the whole genome test could reveal a lot more about a person than just his sporting abilities (25).

GENETIC TESTING FOR INJURY IN SPORTS

This is a new topic in the field of genetics as well. The research, until recently, has focused on how genetic susceptibility could lead to diseases. Now, it is being said that it could lead to sports injuries as well. Meaning that individuals with certain genes could be more susceptible to injuries than others.

One gene which has come up during research is associated with Achilles tendon (AT) and Anterior Cruciate Ligament (ACL) injuries. Recent research suggests the metallo matrix proteins (MMP) are linked to both AT and ACL injuries. The structure of tissues and bones is protected and strengthened by collagen fibres. But in those who are prone to injuries, the collagen fibres to not repair correctly. This problem of collagen not repairing properly is genetically linked. Such individuals are prone to tendinopathy. When a mutation is present in the MMP gene, called the MMP3, and it is linked to the COL5A1 gene, then there is a high risk of such people suffering from tendinopathies, more so if they are an avid athlete who is training hard.

Apart from this, a variation in the COL5A1 gene in South African people was linked to Achilles tendon injuries. There are a few other links with the COL5A1 gene that indicate a person's predisposition to injury. Though no genes have been linked to musculoskeletal injuries, so far.

The cause of injuries can be both extrinsic and intrinsic. Nothing much can be done about intrinsic factors, like genetics, but the extrinsic factors can be controlled. For example, if a person has the gene which could cause tendinopathy, they may possibly look at selecting their primary sport carefully.

Genetics has its advantages and limitations. These should be kept in mind before analyzing the results or predicting a predisposition. When a genetic test is done, the person's family history, medical history, geographical location, environment, and profession should be taken into account. Tests are being designed, and clinicians are being trained to use these tests as and when needed. As always, there are ethical issues related to this (29).

THE LIMIT

How far and how high can humans go? There are many factors involved; biochemical, physical, genetic, dietary, physiological, economic, and environmental to name but a few. With each factor varying for each and every individual, it is difficult to predict an individuals potential.

It was once thought impossible to run one mile in less than 4 minutes, which now seems like a foolish thought since the current world record is 3 minutes and 43 seconds. We can now imagine the situation of the times when people thought this to be impossible. What perceives as impossible now may well be possible in the decades to come.

Some argue that diet and environment play a huge role. Others suggest that diet and environment were actually better in the past, particularly the former where less sugar and fat was consumed. Training equipment and machinery have played a big role. Methodology has improved tremendously. Professionalism also matters. (31)

Another example would be the 800m race, as it was considered absolutely impossible to run sub 1:40 seconds. Currently this record has not been broken, however David Rudisha has come within $1/10^{th}$ of a second . In the last 100 years, the record has decreased in time by nearly exactly 10 seconds (30).

Many sports are going to extreme lengths to progress, team Sky would be an apt example. Swim suits are stitched with laser precision, to avoid the weight of threads and reduce the drag to improve buoyancy and trip of individuals, notably many of these full body swim suits have been banned.

Most genetic studies to-date have been completed on a very small population size. There has been very little variation in the type of athletes involved in these studies too. Replication studies fail many times. These factors make it a little difficult to conclude the findings with certainty.   The genomic revolution is generally focusing on data that can predict life concerns such as diseases. It is however inevitable that a small minority will use this to their advantage.

REFERENCES

1.Forget training those 'muscles': train your 'mitochondria'
10TuesdayDec 2013.
posted by the5krunner in Cycling, Physiology &
Anatomy,Training & Interval Training.

2. Mitochondrial DNA and Maximum Oxygen Consumption.
Matthew B Brearley, Shi Zhou.School of Exercise Science and
Sport Management, Southern Cross University, Lismore, NSW
2480, Australia. Sportscience 5(2), sportsci.org/jour/0102/mbb.htm,
2001 (1775 words).

3. http://www.runningforfitness.org/faq/vo2-max

4. ACE Genetics and V?o2max. Joyner, Michael J.

5. J Appl Physiol (1985). 2000 Mar;88(3):1029-35. Angiotensin-
converting enzyme ID polymorphism and fitness phenotype in the
HERITAGE Family Study. Rankinen T[1], Pérusse L, Gagnon
J, Chagnon YC, Leon AS, Skinner JS, Wilmore JH, Rao
DC, Bouchard C.

6. J Appl Physiol (1985). 1998 Nov;85(5):1842-6. VO2 max is
associated with ACE genotype in postmenopausal women.
Hagberg JM[1], Ferrell RE, McCole SD, Wilund KR, Moore GE.

7. Sports Med. 2013 Sep;43(9):803-17. doi: 10.1007/s40279-013-
0059-4. Genes for elite power and sprint performance: ACTN3
leads the way. Eynon N[1], Hanson ED, Lucia A, Houweling
PJ, Garton F, North KN, Bishop DJ.

8. Similarity of polygenic profiles limits the potential for elite
human physical performance. Alun G. Williams,Jonathan P.
Folland.

9.http://www.theguardian.com/commentisfree/2014/jul/21/jamaicans-sprinting-athletics-commonwealth-games

10.http://www.science20.com/news_articles/genetics_matter_sorry_malcolm_gladwell_you_will_not_be_usain_bolt_no_matter_how_hard_you_practice-139452

11. http://www.news.com.au/sport/commonwealth-games/958-reasons-usain-bolt-is-the-worlds-fastest-man/news-story/33edf559786bf1a4c64b4a272b9e51a8

12. http://www.abc.net.au/radionational/programs/bodysphere/features/4960990

13. http://www.businessinsider.in/16-Revelations-About-Sports-And-Genetics-From-The-Book-That-Destroys-The-10000-Hour-Rule/16-100-years-ago-scientists-believed-that-the-most-average-body-type-was-the-best-body-type-for-athletics/slideshow/21921528.cms

14. https://www.geneticliteracyproject.org/2015/05/20/sports-genes-what-makes-great-athletes-and-why-it-matters/

15. http://www.runhilaryrun.ca/Images/LA_TH_VO2.pdf

16. http://www.pponline.co.uk/encyc/0524.htm#

17. http://www.aemma.org/misc/lactate_threshold.htm

18. http://www.quickanddirtytips.com/health-fitness/exercise/how-to-increase-your-lung-capacity

19. http://www.sentientdevelopments.com/2008/08/michael-phelps-natural-transhuman.html

20. http://www.theguardian.com/sport/blog/2015/apr/19/paula-radcliffe-london-marathon-rousing-send-off-final-race

21. http://www.bbc.co.uk/blogs/gordonfarquhar/2009/08/this_must_be_an_awful.html

22. http://www.usnews.com/science/articles/2009/09/14/when-someone-is-raised-female-and-the-genes-say-xy

23. http://www.washingtonpost.com/wp-dyn/content/article/2008/08/21/AR2008082103680.html

24. http://www.ncbi.nlm.nih.gov/pubmed/15157120

25. http://science.howstuffworks.com/life/genetic/gene-doping1.htm

26. http://news.discovery.com/human/genetics/genetic-testing-for-tomorrows-sports-superstars-151116.htm

27. http://www.smh.com.au/technology/sci-tech/thumbs-down-for-genetic-testing-of-children-for-sports-and-athletic-prowess-20151116-gl06x4.html

28. https://www.hgsa.org.au/documents/item/19

29. http://lermagazine.com/cover_story/genetics-the-future-of-injury-prevention

30. http://sportsscientists.com/2010/11/the-limit-of-human-performance-how-much-faster/

31. http://theconversation.com/is-there-a-limit-to-athletic-performance-8073

www.ingramcontent.com/pod-product-compliance
Lightning Source LLC
Chambersburg PA
CBHW071831200526
45169CB00018B/1342